Read	Trace	
a uma		
I Eu		
am sou		
an uma		
as como		
at às		

Read and write the sentence!

a	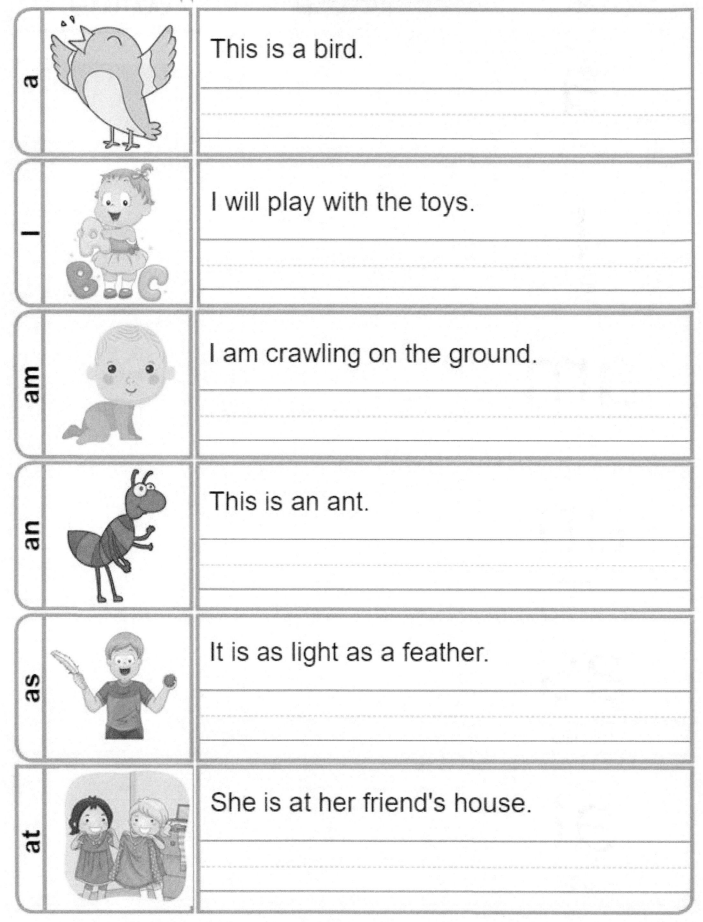	This is a bird.
I		I will play with the toys.
am		I am crawling on the ground.
an		This is an ant.
as		It is as light as a feather.
at		She is at her friend's house.

Read	Trace	Write

be
estar

by
de

do
faz

go
vai

he
ele

if
e se

Read and write the sentence!

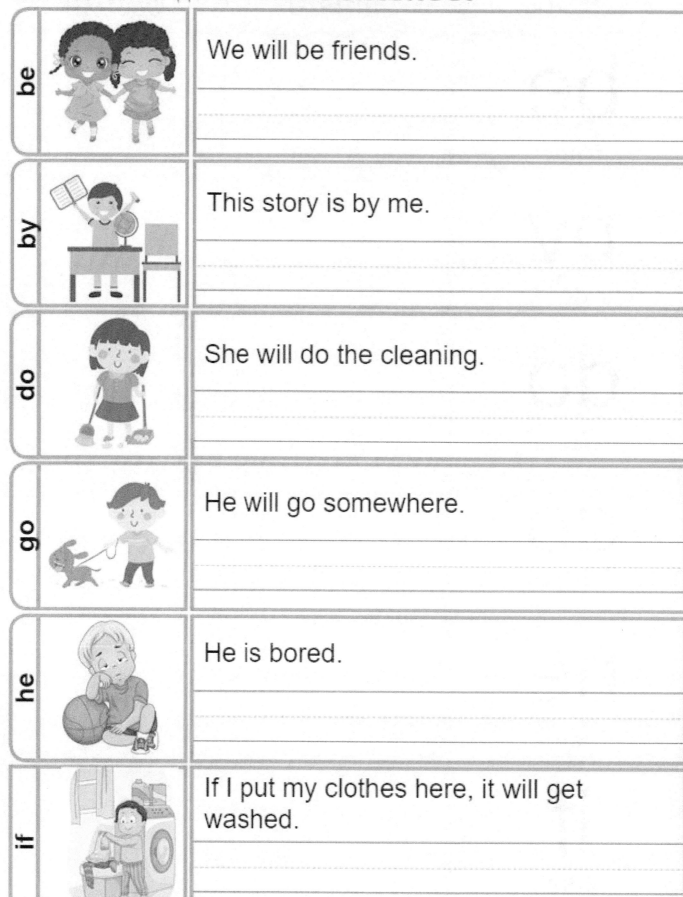

be — We will be friends.

by — This story is by me.

do — She will do the cleaning.

go — He will go somewhere.

he — He is bored.

if — If I put my clothes here, it will get washed.

Read	Trace	Write
in no		
is é		
it isto		
me mim		
my meu		
no não		

Read and write the sentence!

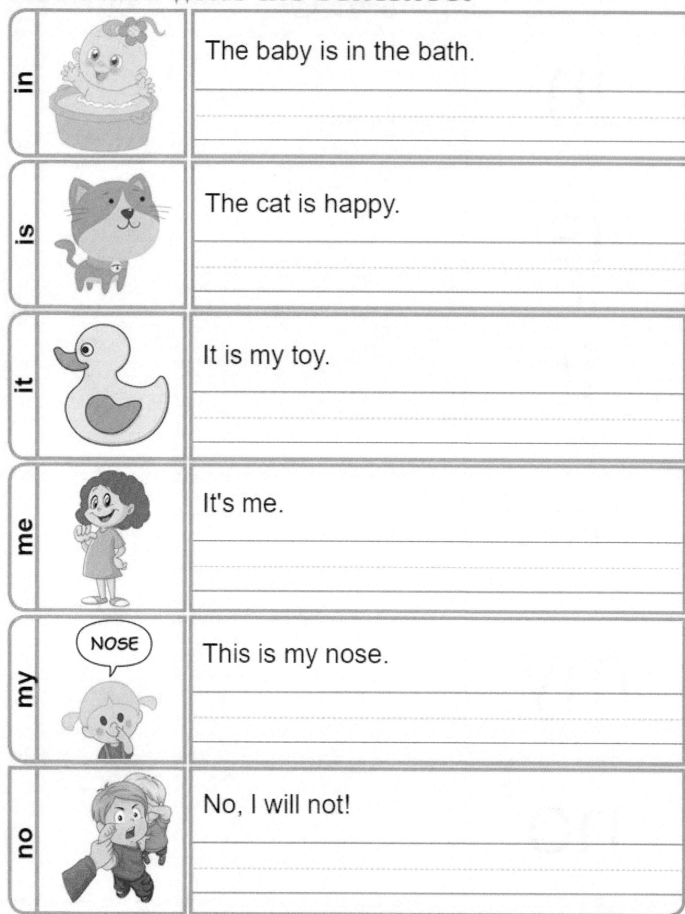

in	The baby is in the bath.
is	The cat is happy.
it	It is my toy.
me	It's me.
my	This is my nose.
no	No, I will not!

Read	Trace	Write

of
do

on
em

or
ou

so
tão

to
para

up
acima

Read and write the sentence!

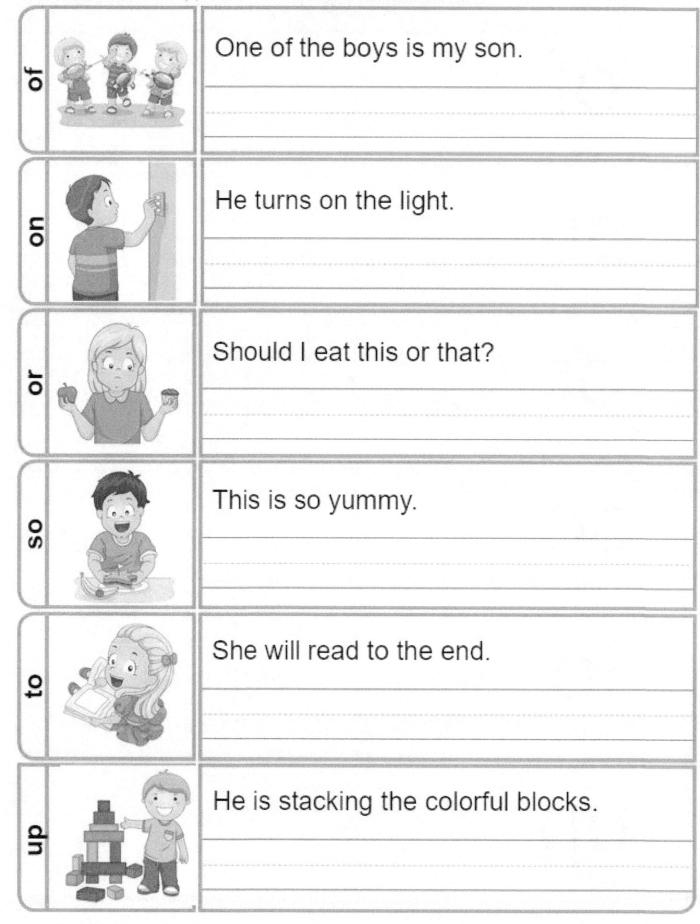

of — One of the boys is my son.

on — He turns on the light.

or — Should I eat this or that?

so — This is so yummy.

to — She will read to the end.

up — He is stacking the colorful blocks.

Read	Trace	Write
us nos		
we nós		
all todos		
and e		
any qualquer		
are estamos		

Read and write the sentence!

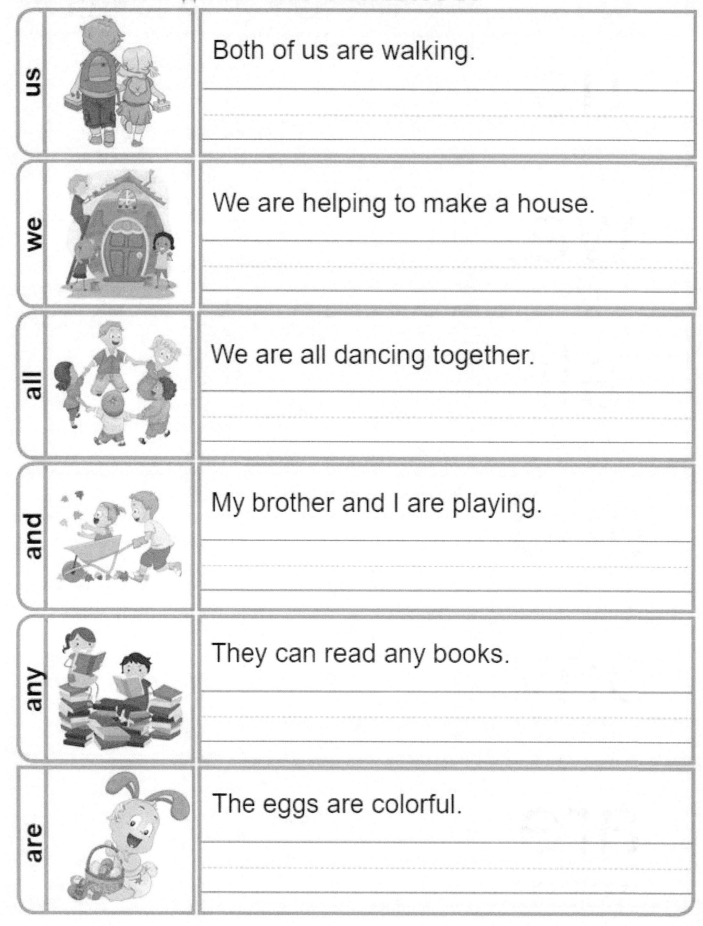

us — Both of us are walking.

we — We are helping to make a house.

all — We are all dancing together.

and — My brother and I are playing.

any — They can read any books.

are — The eggs are colorful.

Read	Trace	Write
ask perguntar		
ate comeu		
bed cama		
big grande		
box caixa		
boy garoto		

Read and write the sentence!

ask	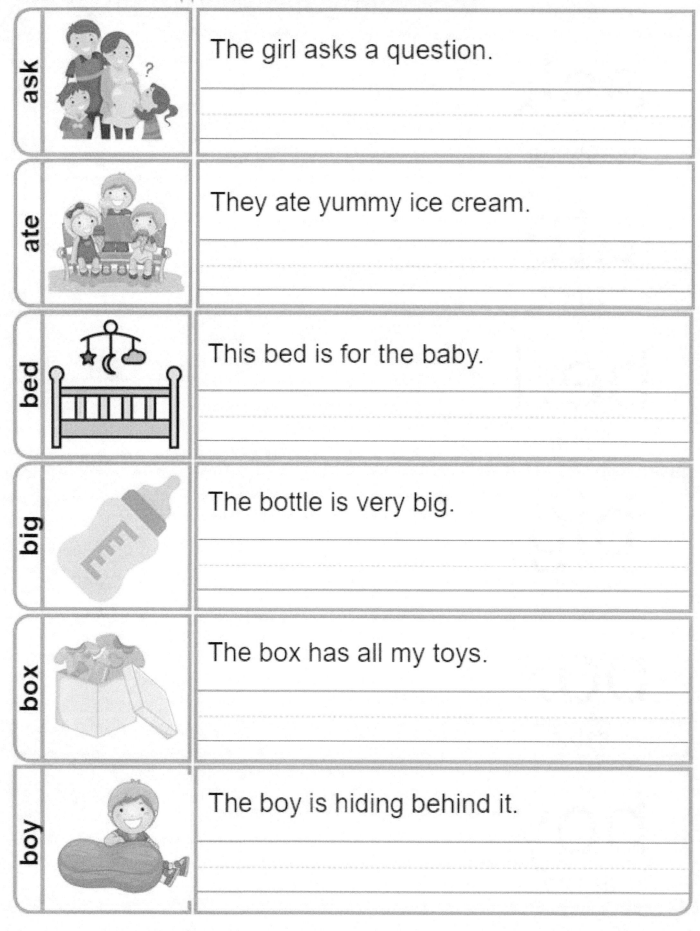	The girl asks a question.
ate		They ate yummy ice cream.
bed		This bed is for the baby.
big		The bottle is very big.
box		The box has all my toys.
boy		The boy is hiding behind it.

Read	Trace	Write
but mas		
buy comprar		
can lata		
car carro		
cat gato		
cow vaca		

Read and write the sentence!

but	I want to go, but my son doesn't.
buy	He buys lots of stuff.
can	The baby will drink milk from the can.
car	The car is red.
cat	The cat is sad.
cow	The cow is funny.

Read	Trace	Write
cut cortar		
day dia		
did fez		
dog cão		
eat comer		
egg ovo		

Read and write the sentence!

cut		They are cutting out paper.
day	Month 30	This day is the 30th.
did		She did a great job.
dog		The dog is adorable.
eat		The monkey will eat the banana.
egg		The egg is small.

Read	Trace	Write
eye olho		
far longe		
fly mosca		
for para		
get pegue		
got obteve		

Read and write the sentence!

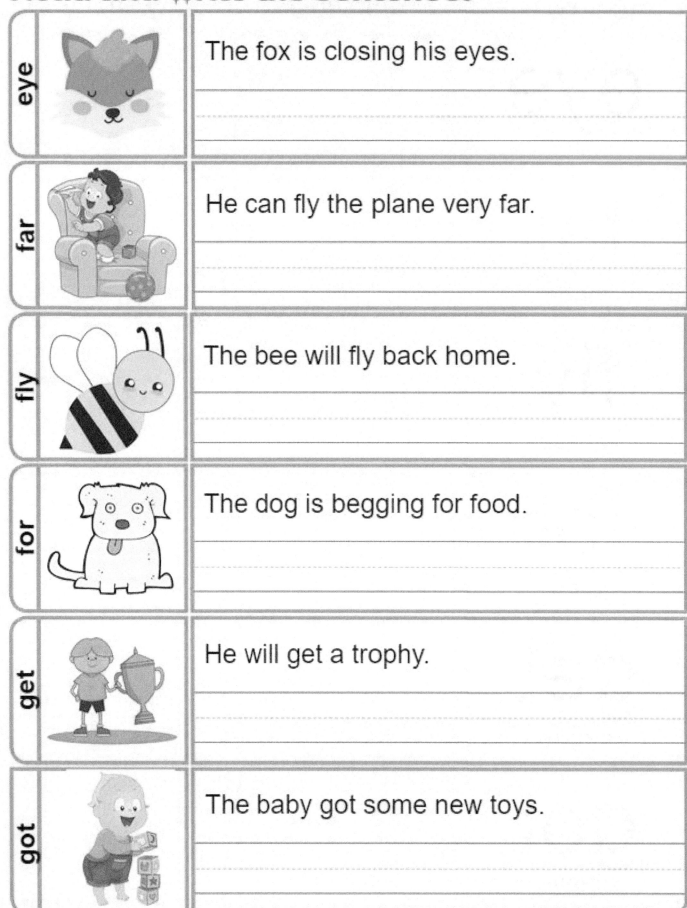

eye — The fox is closing his eyes.

far — He can fly the plane very far.

fly — The bee will fly back home.

for — The dog is begging for food.

get — He will get a trophy.

got — The baby got some new toys.

Read	Trace	Write
had teve		
has tem		
her dela		
him ele		
his seu		
hot quente		

Read and write the sentence!

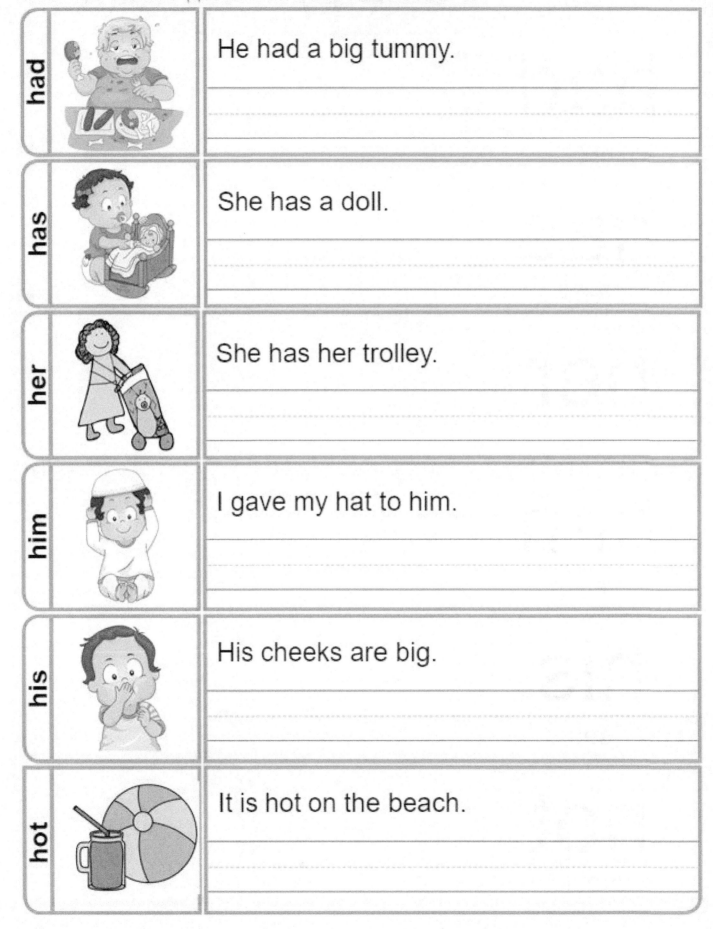

had — He had a big tummy.

has — She has a doll.

her — She has her trolley.

him — I gave my hat to him.

his — His cheeks are big.

hot — It is hot on the beach.

Read	Trace	Write

how
como

its
está

leg
perna

let
deixei

man
cara

may
maio

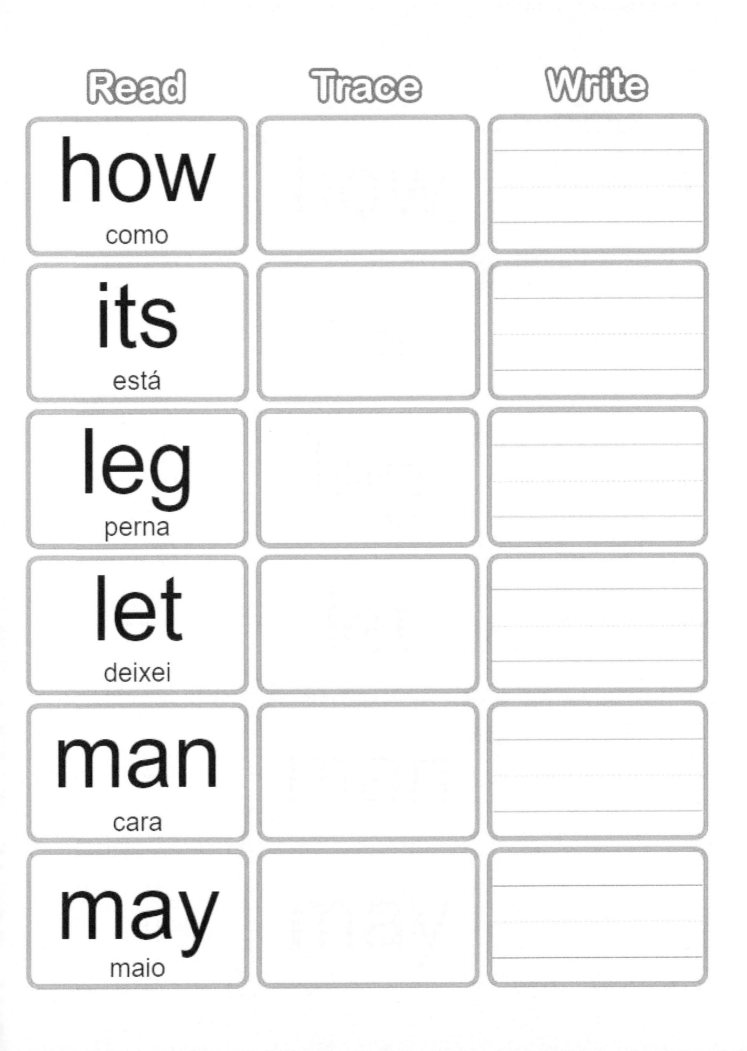

Read and write the sentence!

how		How many blocks are there?
its		Its legs are short.
leg		His legs are short.
let		Let me come in!
man		The man is a vet.
may		May I have more?

Read	Trace	Write
men homens		
new novo		
not não		
now agora		
off fora		
old velho		

Read and write the sentence!

men		The men are mining for gold.
new		She has a new hat.
not		She is not feeling well.
now		Now I am doing my homework.
off		They cut off the paper.
old		You are one year old!

Read	Trace	Write
one uma		
our nosso		
out fora		
own próprio		
pig porco		
put colocar		

Read and write the sentence!

one	The panda says one.
our	This is our room.
out	He will go out.
own	The man owns a computer.
pig	She is sleeping on her pig.
put	She is putting an arm around her daughter.

Read	Trace	Write
ran corre		
red vermelho		
run corre		
saw vejo		
say dizer		
see vejo		

Read and write the sentence!

ran		She ran back home.
red		The bus is red.
run		He is running away from the bats.
saw		He saw something.
say		You should always say Please.
see		They see something in the sky.

Read	Trace	Write

she
ela

sit
sentar

six
seis

sun
sol

ten
dez

the
1

Read and write the sentence!

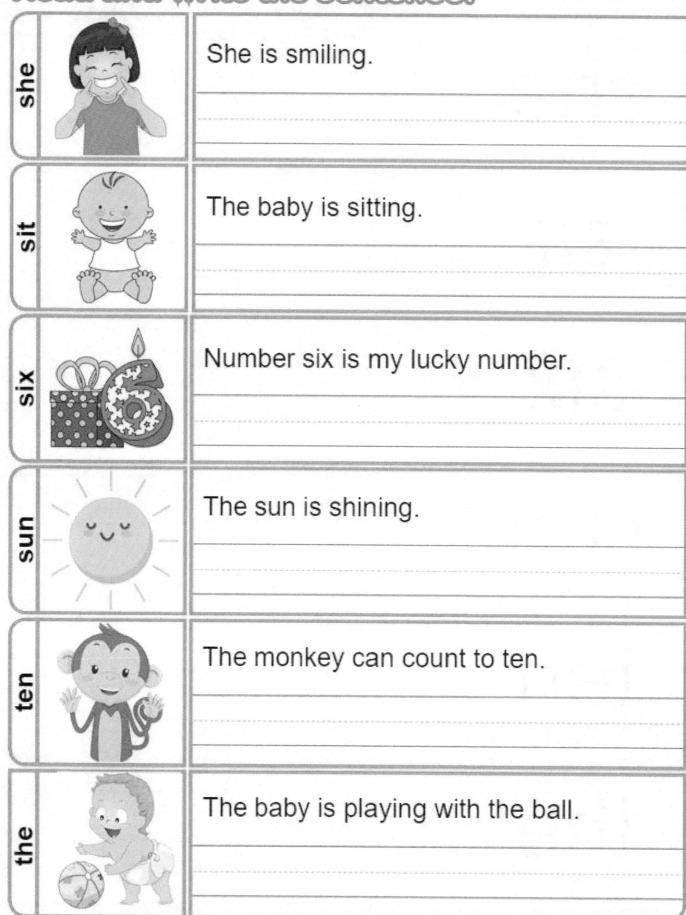

she		She is smiling.
sit		The baby is sitting.
six		Number six is my lucky number.
sun		The sun is shining.
ten		The monkey can count to ten.
the		The baby is playing with the ball.

Read	Trace	Write

too
também

top
topo

toy
brinquedo

try
tentar

two
dois

use
usar

Read and write the sentence!

too	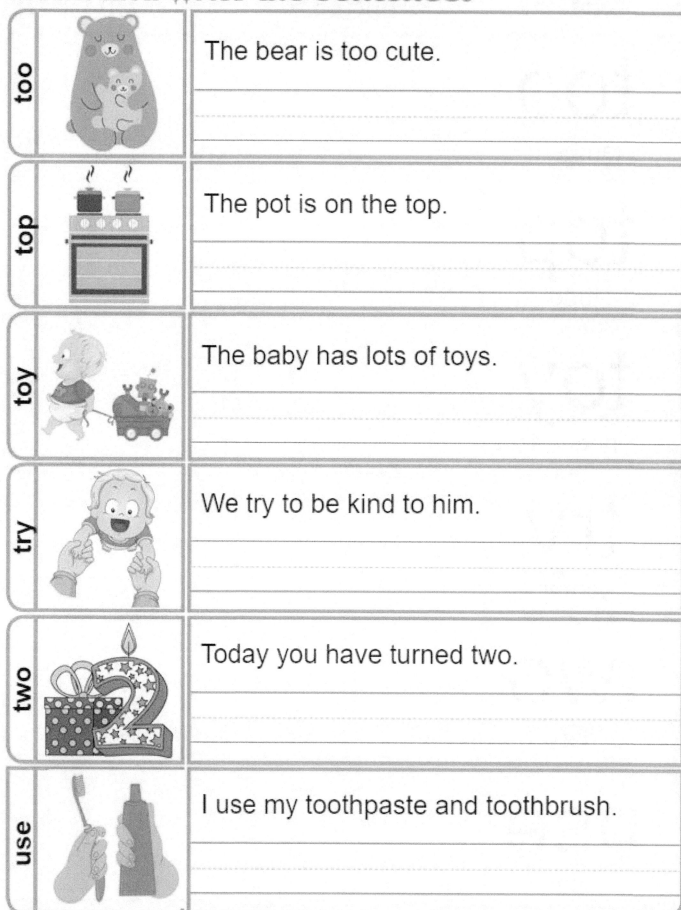	The bear is too cute.
top		The pot is on the top.
toy		The baby has lots of toys.
try		We try to be kind to him.
two		Today you have turned two.
use		I use my toothpaste and toothbrush.

Read	Trace	Write
was foi		
way caminho		
who o que		
why porque		
yes sim		
you você		

Read and write the sentence!

was	He was reading a book.
way	Let's go this way
who	Who wants to dance?
why	Why is the machine not working?
yes	Yes, I am so happy!
you	I love you!

Read	Trace	Write
away longe		
baby bebê		
back de volta		
ball bola		
bear urso		
been foi		

Read and write the sentence!

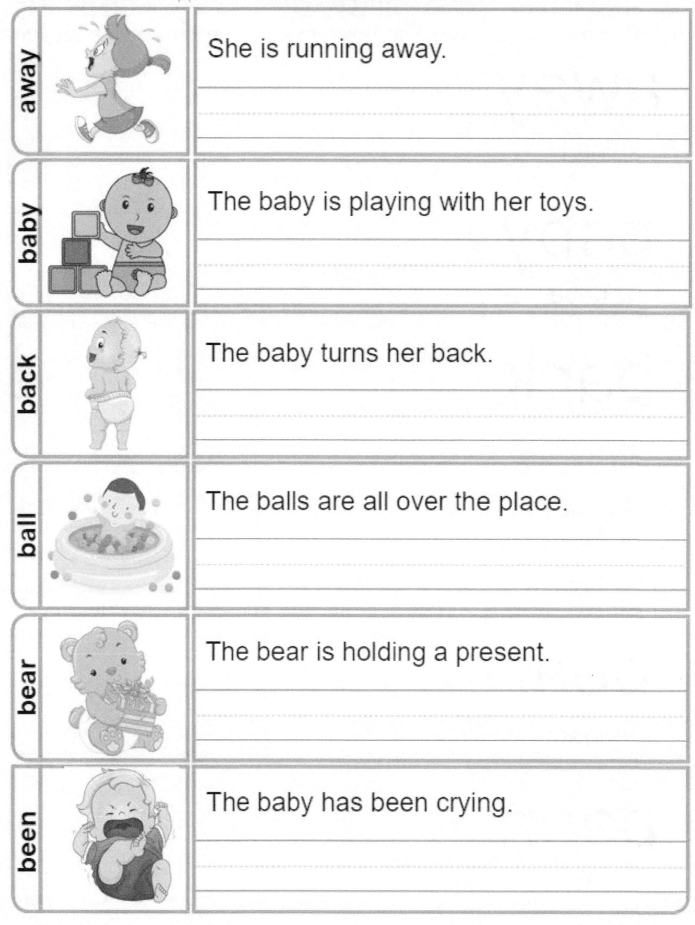

away		She is running away.
baby		The baby is playing with her toys.
back		The baby turns her back.
ball		The balls are all over the place.
bear		The bear is holding a present.
been		The baby has been crying.

Read	Trace	Write

bell
sino

best
melhor

bird
pássaro

blue
azul

boat
barco

both
ambos

Read and write the sentence!

bell		The bells are ringing.
best		This is the best food for babies.
bird		The bird is flying.
blue		The boy dressed up in blue.
boat		The boat will go into the ocean.
both		Both of you look so much alike.

Read	Trace	Write

cake
bolo

call
ligar

came
veio

coat
casaco

cold
frio

come
venha

Read and write the sentence!

cake		The cake is for your birthday.
call		She is calling for somebody.
came		She came with her bag.
coat		The girl is wearing her coat.
cold		The baby feels cold.
come		Come here to the slide!

Read	Trace	Write
corn milho		
does faz		
doll boneca		
done feito		
door porta		
down baixa		

Read and write the sentence!

corn		The corn tastes good.
does		Does that thing taste bad?
doll		She is hugging her doll.
done		I've done reading my book.
door		They open the door.
down		The boy turns his head down.

Read	Trace	Write
draw desenhar		
duck pato		
fall outono		
farm fazenda		
fast velozes		
feet pé		

Read and write the sentence!

draw	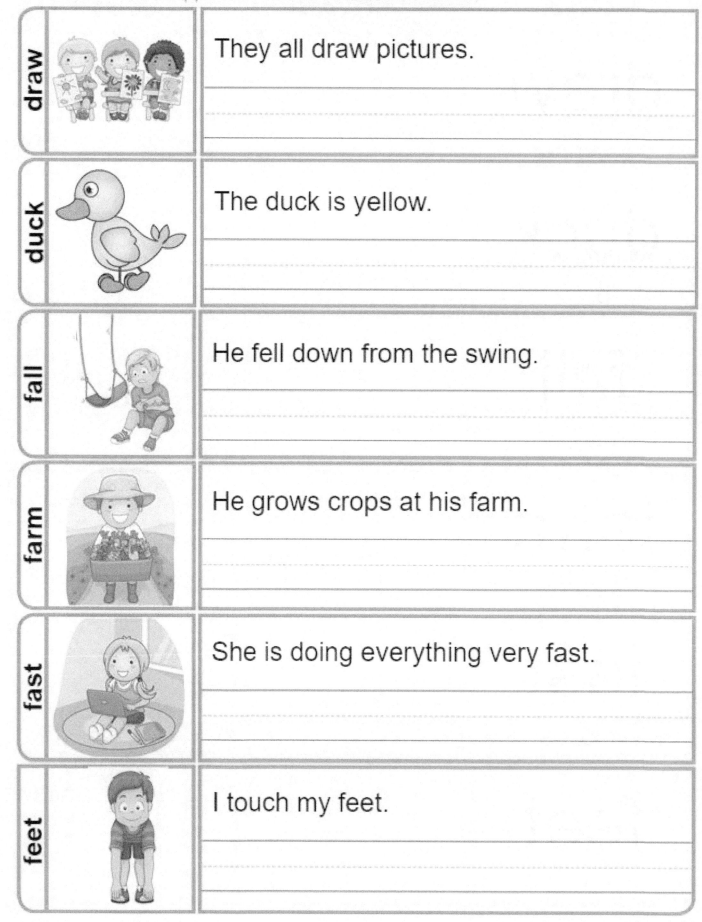	They all draw pictures.
duck		The duck is yellow.
fall		He fell down from the swing.
farm		He grows crops at his farm.
fast		She is doing everything very fast.
feet		I touch my feet.

Read	Trace	Write
find encontrar		
fire fogo		
fish peixe		
five cinco		
four quatro		
from de		

Read and write the sentence!

find	They are finding something.
fire	The fire is blazing and dangerous.
fish	The fish are swimming in the ocean.
five	You get birthday gifts for turning five.
four	The lion is turning four today.
from	She will draw a picture of her flower.

Read	Trace	Write
full cheio		
game jogos		
gave deu		
girl menina		
give dar		
goes vai		

Read and write the sentence!

full	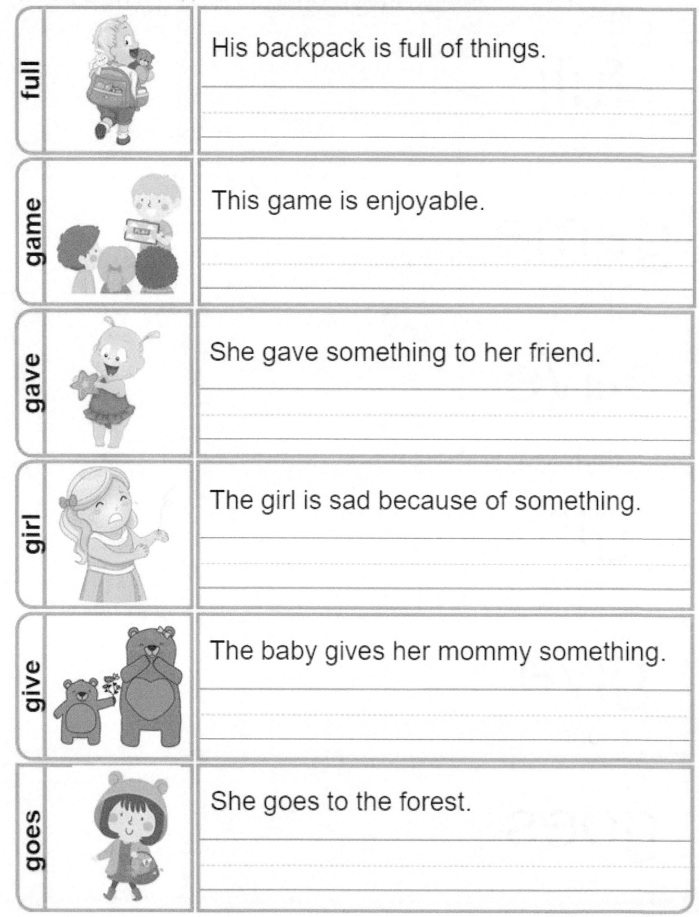	His backpack is full of things.
game		This game is enjoyable.
gave		She gave something to her friend.
girl		The girl is sad because of something.
give		The baby gives her mommy something.
goes		She goes to the forest.

Read	Trace	Write
good boa		
grow crescer		
hand mão		
have ter		
head cabeça		
help socorro		

Read and write the sentence!

good		The baby is acting very well today.
grow		My plant will grow!
hand		My hand is touching the wall.
have		She will have lots of friends.
head	HEAD	My head is round.
help		They help each other wash the clothes.

Read	Trace	Write
here aqui		
hill colina		
hold aguarde		
home casa		
hurt doeu		
into para dentro		

Read and write the sentence!

here		America is over here.
hill		The hill has some trees and a house.
hold		He is holding his daughter.
home		He drew a picture of his home.
hurt		The boy is hurt.
into		He will jump into the pool.

Read	Trace	Write
jump saltar		
just somente		
keep guarda		
kind tipo		
know conhecer		
like gostar		

Read and write the sentence!

jump	The cat jumped on the cushion.
just	The arrival of the plane just arrived.
keep	She keeps thinking about it.
kind	The woman is kind to the girl.
know	They know that they will go over there.
like	He likes to ride on the horse.

Read	Trace	Write
live viver		
long longo		
look veja		
made fez		
make fez		
many muitos		

Read and write the sentence!

live		They all live together.
long		The pencil is very long.
look		They are looking at something.
made		They made a promise.
make		They are going to make something.
many		He has many shirts.

Read	Trace	Write
milk leite		
much muito de		
must devo		
name nome		
nest ninho		
once uma vez		

Read and write the sentence!

milk	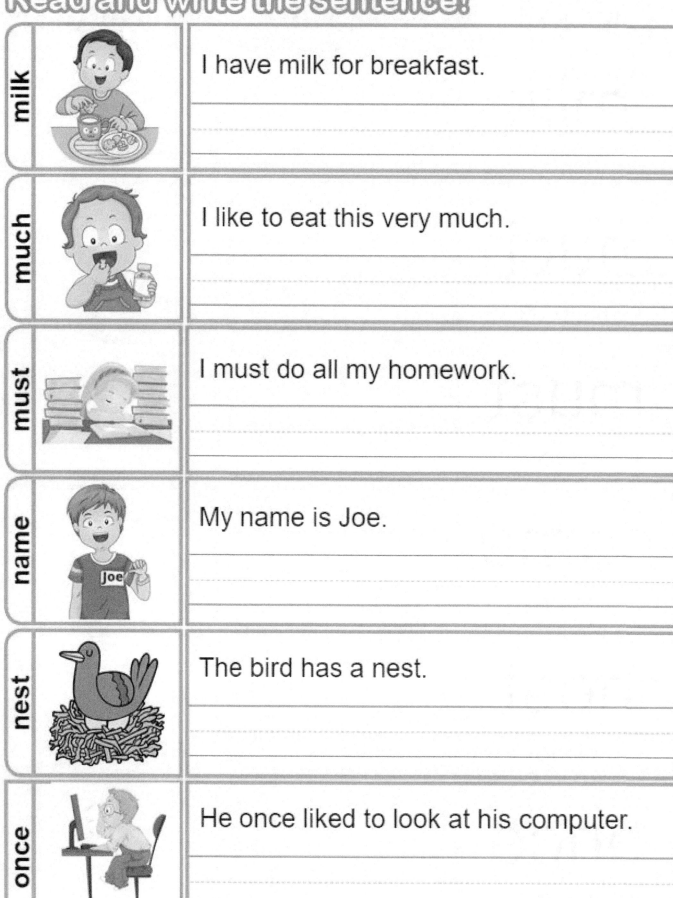	I have milk for breakfast.
much		I like to eat this very much.
must		I must do all my homework.
name		My name is Joe.
nest		The bird has a nest.
once		He once liked to look at his computer.

Read	Trace	Write
only só		
open aberto		
over sobre		
pick escolher		
play toque		
pull puxar		

Read and write the sentence!

only	There is only one student.
open	He wants to open the door.
over	The class is over.
pick	She picked up something.
play	They like to play together.
pull	She is pulling on her friend's hair.

Read	Trace	Write
rain chuva		
read ler		
ride passeio		
ring anel		
said disse		
seed semente		

Read and write the sentence!

rain		The rain is not going to hit us.
read		She likes to read books.
ride		The baby is riding on a toy horse.
ring		The bird is holding a ring in its beak.
said		She said hello to her neighbor.
seed	SEEDS	The seeds are going to plant.

Read	Trace	Write
shoe sapato		
show exposição		
sing cantar		
snow neve		
some alguns		
song canção		

Read and write the sentence!

shoe		Her shoes are cute and purple.
show		This map shows the location.
sing		The baby can sing along.
snow		I like to play snow.
some		These are some of my toys.
song		I will sing a song in the talent show.

Read	Trace	Write
soon em breve		
stop pare		
take toma		
tell contar		
that aquele		
them eles		

Read and write the sentence!

soon	The eggs will hatch soon.
stop	The teacher says to stop.
take	They take some flowers.
tell	She is telling a story.
that	That bird dressed up as Santa.
them	He likes to eat them.

Read	Trace	Write
then então		
they eles		
this isto		
time tempo		
tree árvore		
upon em cima de		

Read and write the sentence!

then		Then, I will go to bed.
they		They are running to school.
this		This is my duck.
time		The time always moves on.
tree		There are lots of green trees in the park.
upon		Once upon a time, there was a princess.

Read	Trace	Write
very muito		
walk andar		
want quer		
warm caloroso		
wash lavar		
well bem		

Read and write the sentence!

very	The baby is lovely.
walk	They are walking on the sidewalk.
want	The baby wants more milk.
warm	The bath is warm.
wash	She is going to wash the dishes.
well	He can save money well.

Read	Trace	Write
went foi		
were estamos		
what o que		
when quando		
will vai		
wind vento		

Read and write the sentence!

went		The crocodile went to the pond.
were		There were lots of toys.
what		What is the lion doing?
when		When are you going to wake up?
will		Will I get it in?
wind		The wind is blowing fiercely.

Read	Trace	Write
wish desejo		
with com		
wood madeira		
work trabalhos		
your seu		
about sobre		

Read and write the sentence!

wish		I wish you a happy Christmas!
with		He is with his sister.
wood		He is stacking up wooden blocks.
work		He is going to work in his tractor.
your		Your baby is wearing a yellow suit.
about		It's about to be 12:30.

Read	Trace	Write
after depois de		
again novamente		
apple maçã		
black preto		
bread pão		
bring trazer		

Read and write the sentence!

after		The teacher calmed them after they fought.
again		He did it again!
apple		The apple is red and juicy.
black		The crow is black.
bread		My breakfast is bread and jam.
bring		He is bringing his project.

Read	Trace	Write
brown castanho		
carry levar		
chair cadeira		
clean limpo		
could lata		
don't não		

Read and write the sentence!

brown		Her stuffed animal is a brown bear.
carry		He is carrying a big crayon.
chair		He is sitting on his chair.
clean		He needs to clean up.
could		The baby could do push-ups.
don't		Don't do that!

Read	Trace	Write
drink bebida		
eight oito		
every cada		
first primeiro		
floor chão		
found encontrado		

Read and write the sentence!

drink	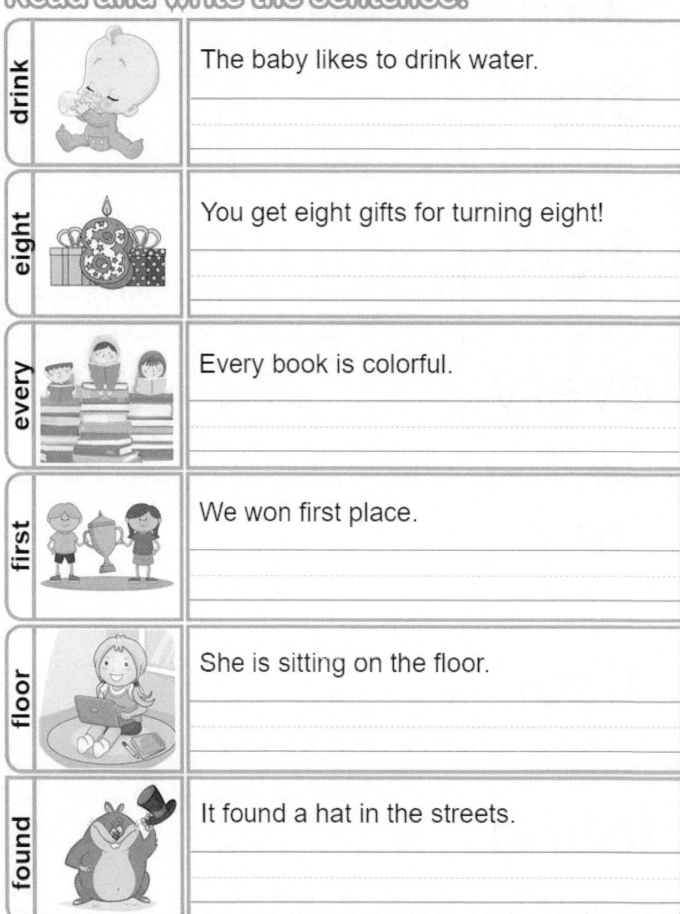	The baby likes to drink water.
eight		You get eight gifts for turning eight!
every		Every book is colorful.
first		We won first place.
floor		She is sitting on the floor.
found		It found a hat in the streets.

Read	Trace	Write

funny
engraçado

going
vai

grass
relva

green
verde

horse
cavalo

house
casa

Read and write the sentence!

funny		The rabbit thinks the joke is funny.
going		The bear is going to eat all the honey.
grass		The goat eats grass on the hill.
green		The turtle that is walking is green.
horse		The horse is magical.
house		They lived in that house.

Read	Trace	Write
kitty gato		
laugh rir		
light leve		
money dinheiro		
never nunca		
night noite		

Read and write the sentence!

kitty	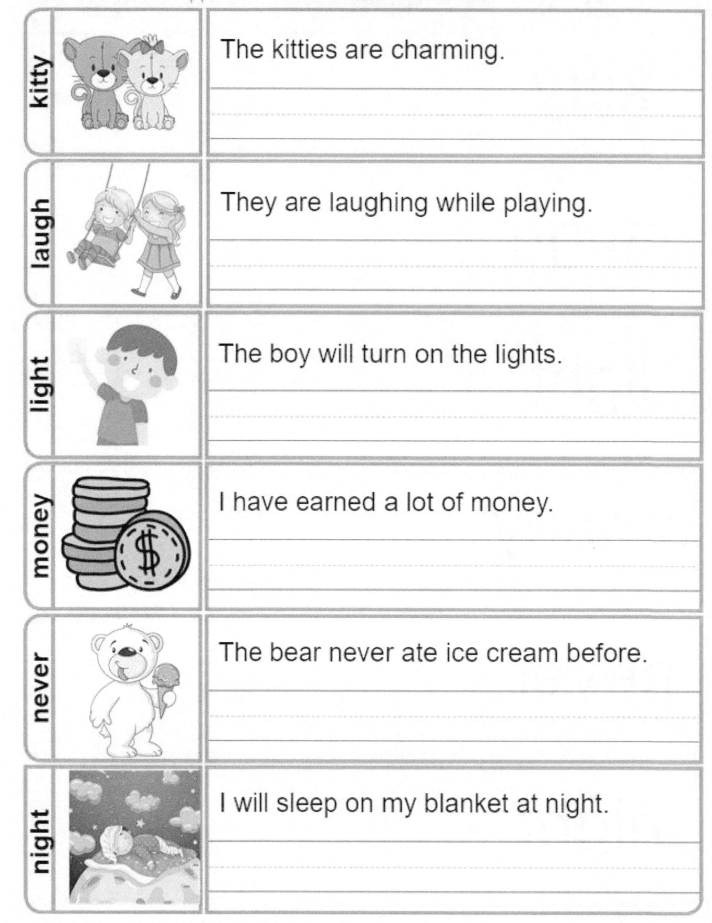	The kitties are charming.
laugh		They are laughing while playing.
light		The boy will turn on the lights.
money		I have earned a lot of money.
never		The bear never ate ice cream before.
night		I will sleep on my blanket at night.

Read	Trace	Write
paper papel		
party festa		
right corrigir		
round volta		
seven sete		
shall deve		

Read and write the sentence!

paper		I will draw on the paper for a project.
party		The party will be for her birthday.
right		They say we have to go right.
round		The frogs' eyes are round.
seven		The monkey can count to seven.
shall		Shall I make a garden?

Read	Trace	Write
sheep ovelha		
sleep dormir		
small pequeno		
start começar		
stick gravetos		
table mesa		

Read and write the sentence!

sheep		The sheep have a bell around its neck.
sleep		I will go to sleep in my comfortable bed.
small		The small baby will crawl to its crib.
start		She will start sleeping soon.
stick		He has some sticks to play.
table		The table has a toy on it.

Read	Trace	Write
thank obrigado		
their deles		
there há		
these estes		
thing coisa		
think pensar		

Read and write the sentence!

thank	He made a Thank you card for you.
their	They will enjoy their picnic.
there	There is something in front of you.
these	These are my eating material.
thing	The thing is broken.
think	She thinks about what she is going to draw.

Read	Trace	Write
those essa		
three três		
today hoje		
under debaixo		
watch ver		
water água		

Read and write the sentence!

those		Those are mine.
three		She will turn three today.
today		Today is a beautiful day.
under		The puppy sleeps under the blanket.
watch		They both watch the video.
water		He is drinking water after a long soccer game.

Read	Trace	Write
where onde		
which qual		
white branco		
would seria		
write escreva		
always sempre		

Read and write the sentence!

where	Where are we?
which	The clothes which are my sisters are colorful.
white	The sheep have white wool.
would	He would tell them a story.
write	I like to write lots of stories.
always	I am always happy that it is Christmas.

Read	Trace	Write
around por aí		
before antes		
better melhor		
farmer agricultor		
father pai		
flower flor		

Read and write the sentence!

around		I will shuffle the shapes around.
before		Before I go to school, I kiss my mom.
better		I can make it better.
farmer		The farmer takes care of the animals.
father		My father is wearing a blue shirt.
flower		She will play with the flowers.

Read	Trace	Write
garden jardim		
ground terra		
letter cartas		
little pouco		
mother mãe		
myself eu mesmo		

Read and write the sentence!

garden		Her garden is vast and healthy.
ground		I am playing with my dog on the ground.
letter		These are the letters A, B, and C.
little		The world is small.
mother		My mother is very nice.
myself		I made these by myself.

Read	Trace	Write
please por favor		
pretty bonita		
rabbit coelho		
school escola		
sister irmã		
street rua		

Read and write the sentence!

please	Please stop pulling my hair.
pretty	She made the cake very pretty.
rabbit	The rabbit is white and soft.
school	This is the school.
sister	My sister is wearing a pink dress.
street	They are walking across the street.

Read	Trace	Write
window janela		
yellow amarelo		
because porque		
brother irmão		
chicken frango		
goodbye tchau		

Read and write the sentence!

window		The window is open.
yellow		The ducky is yellow.
because		She will sleep because it is night.
brother		His brother is playing with him.
chicken		The chicken has hatched out of the egg.
goodbye		The animal is saying goodbye.

Read	Trace	Write
morning manhã		
picture cenário		
birthday aniversário		
children crianças		
squirrel esquilo		
together juntos		

Read and write the sentence!

morning		He likes to ride his bike in the morning.
picture		He will take a picture.
birthday		Today is my birthday!
children		The children are doing something.
squirrel		The squirrel is cute.
together		They are sharing a bed together.

Made in the USA
Columbia, SC
27 March 2025

55762568R00059